Apple Cider Vinegar for Beginners:

Weight Loss, Recipes, Remedies & Miracle Cures for a Healthy, Happy Life

Table of Contents

Copyright

terms of inattention or otherwise, by any usage or abuse of any policies, processes, or directions contained within is the solitary and utter responsibility of the recipient reader. Under no circumstances will any legal responsibility or blame be held against the publisher for any reparation, damages, or monetary loss due to the information herein, either directly or indirectly.

Respective authors own all copyrights not held by the publisher.

The information herein is offered for informational purposes solely, and is universal as so. The presentation of the information is without contract or any type of guarantee assurance.

The trademarks that are used are without any consent, and the publication of the trademark is without permission or backing by the trademark owner. All trademarks and brands within this book are for clarifying purposes only and are the owned by the owners themselves, not affiliated with this document.

Introduction

Apple Cider Vinegar (ACV) is known not only for making recipes taste better but also for its healing properties. Apple cider vinegar offers a lot of benefits ranging from weight loss to health and beauty remedies.

In this book, you will learn:

- How to use apple cider vinegar to lose weight effectively
- How to cure various health conditions using ACV
- How to use this miracle vinegar for beauty purposes
- Apple cider vinegar recipes for diet, health remedies and beauty enhancements.

Apple Cider Vinegar is all-natural. It does not contain any harsh preservatives or unhealthy chemicals that can cause health issues.

If you want to live a healthy life using natural means, this book is the best guide you will ever need.

Enjoy!

Chapter 1 Apple Cider Vinegar for Health

Apple cider vinegar is much more than just an addition to your recipes. Due to its antibacterial, antifungal and antiviral properties, apple cider vinegar has been used to relieve various medical conditions by our ancestors.

Check out the list below to learn about the health benefits of ACV:

Diarrhea other stomach issues

This vinegar has antibiotic properties which helps relieve tummy troubles caused by bacteria. Furthermore, apple cider vinegar contains pectin which helps soothe intestinal spasms.
Mix 2 tablespoons ACV in 1 glass of warm water and drink twice a day. This drink will relieve your symptoms quickly.

Sore throat

When your throat starts to feel itchy and sore, apple cider vinegar can help stop the infection. Mix ¼ cup of ACV in 1 glass of lukewarm water and gargle as often as needed. The acetic acid in this vinegar will relieve the itch. On the other hand, its antibacterial properties will prevent bacterial growth. You will feel relief as soon as you are done gargling with this mixture.

Foot Odor and Body Odor

The acids in ACV helps balance the pH level of your skin. As a result, the odor-causing bacteria and germs that cause your underarm and feet smell are eliminated. Soak individual tissue papers, paper towels or baby wipes overnight in apple cider vinegar. Store in an air-tight container or zip lock and keep in the fridge for a day. Use it as needed. Although this vinegar has a strong acidic smell, it does go away when it dries.

Itch Relief

This all-around vinegar is also great for relieving itch caused by insect bites. It also provides great relief for jelly fish sting. Just apply ACV (Apple Cider Vinegar) directly on the affected area and feel relieved instantly.

Lower Cholesterol

In one study, the acetic acid found in apple cider vinegar caused a drop in the bad cholesterol level in lab rats. Another study also showed that apple cider vinegar helps reduce blood pressure in rats. Unfortunately, these results still need to be tested in humans. One Japanese study showed that people who consumed half an ounce of apple cider vinegar everyday has lower cholesterol level. This result still needs to be studied further.

Stuffy Nose

Apple cider vinegar contains potassium which helps thin mucus. It also contains acetic acid that prevents the growth of bacteria, therefore preventing nasal congestion. Mix 1 tablespoon of ACV in a glass of warm water and drink early in the morning and before sleeping to help drain your sinus.

Lower Blood Sugar Level

Drinking apple cider vinegar helps improve insulin sensitivity and lowers blood sugar response during meals. That being said, ACV is beneficial for people with diabetes or for those who are not diabetic but wants to keep their blood sugar levels to normal. Just drink 2 tablespoons of this multi-purpose vinegar before going to bed to reduce your blood sugar by up to 4%.

Weight Loss

The acetic acid found in ACV suppresses your appetite and increases your satiety. Therefore, it makes you feel fuller and lets you eat lesser. Research also suggests that ACV makes you eat lesser calories because it interferes with your body's digestion of starch, resulting to fewer calories entering your bloodstream.

Take 1 tablespoon of apple cider vinegar before each meal to help you reduce weight. You may also combine 3 parts ACV to 1 part olive oil and use it to massage your problem areas to help reduce your body fats.

Energy Drink

If you feel tired or weary or simply out of energy, give yourself a boost by adding 2 tablespoons of apple cider vinegar in a glass of water. You may add a tablespoon of honey for a little bit of sweetness. The enzymes and potassium found in ACV will boost your energy and take you to a higher gear.

Sunburn Relief

If your entire body is affected by sunburn, mix 1 cup of apple cider vinegar in your cool bath water and soak for 15 to 20 minutes.   Pat your body dry and apply ACV directly on needed areas.

Headache

Vaporized ACV works wonders. Add 2 tablespoons of apple cider vinegar in a vaporizer or a pan with purified water. Heat the mixture until it boils. Remove from heat and place a towel over your head and lean on the pan of steaming ACV mixture. Breathe the steam vapors.

Add a cup of raw, undiluted apple cider vinegar in your warm bath. Soak in the warm bath mixture for 15 to 20 minutes. Do this during your morning bath and before going to bed at night.

External Itching

If you are experiencing itch due to allergic reactions, dry skin or imbalance in your body, simply dilute ¼ cup of ACV in 1 cup of water. Soak a cotton ball in the mixture and apply directly on the itch. Use as needed.

Leg Cramps and Swollen Muscles

Mix 2 tablespoons raw ACV in 1 cup of warm water and use it to massage the painful areas. The potassium in ACV will relieve your muscle spasm.

Hiccups

Hiccups can be very annoying and distracting. To get rid of hiccups, drink 1 to 2 tablespoons ACV. You'll be surprised at how fast your hiccups were relieved.

Urinary Tract Infection

Drink 2 tablespoons of ACV in the morning and in the evening. ACV will restore your body's natural pH balance. It will also prevent the growth of bacteria that causes UTI.

Dog Fleas

To fight off those pesky fleas from your dog, add 2 tablespoons of Apple cider vinegar in 1 liter of water and use it as the final rinse during your dog's bath. Your dog will be free from fleas and will have smoother, odor-free hair instantly.

Chapter 2: ACV for Weight Loss

As mentioned in Chapter 1, apple cider vinegar is a great aid in reducing excess body fats. Due to the acetic acid content of this miracle vinegar, your appetite is suppressed and you feel fuller easily. Furthermore, ACV interferes with your body's digestion of starch. As a result, your body absorbs fewer calories.

This transforms to reduced weight and lesser body fats. In addition, ACV contains enzymes that helps boost your metabolism rate. Higher metabolism means more body fats burned. As a result, your body also retains less water, making you feel more energized. Also, ACV lowers blood sugar levels which translate to lesser insulin. Studies show that lower insulin level helps reduce body weight.

Along with healthier food choices and regular exercise, simply add 2 tablespoons of apple cider vinegar in 16 ounces of warm water mixed with 1 tablespoon honey and drink it every day. It is recommended to drink this mixture before each meal. You may also add 2 tablespoons of ACV on your tea with a tablespoon of honey or maple syrup. Remember; do not go beyond 2 tablespoons for every drink. Another tasty option is to add one to two tablespoons of Apple Cider Vinegar on your daily smoothie. This way, you are able to incorporate ACV in your diet without even realizing it.

Since apple cider vinegar is an all-natural product, it does not have any harmful side effects and you can take it for as long as you want. But of course, anything that is too much is harmful, so stick to 2 tablespoons per drinking session only. Also, the effect of apple cider vinegar on weight loss is not immediate and it varies depending on your body type. Some have lost 2 pounds in 3 weeks while others lost 4 pounds in a month.

For a more effective weight loss using apple cider vinegar, you can add banana to your diet as it contains potassium which lowers blood pressure. Banana is also known to reduce stress. Additionally, cut down your sugar intake as it can spike insulin levels. It will also help if you exercise more. For instance, you can have a 30-minute walk every day or go biking during weekends.

Chapter 3: Apple Cider Vinegar for Beauty

Apple cider vinegar has a lot of benefits. It is a natural product that helps keep bacteria and germs away from your body. Not only is ACV beneficial to your health, it can also help you have better skin, get away with warts and much more.

Dandruff Remover

Due to the antifungal properties of this vinegar, the fungus that causes the growth of dandruff is eliminated. Mix ¼ cup of apple cider vinegar in ¼ cup of water and place it in a spray container. Spray this mixture on your scalp after you shampoo. Let it stay on your scalp for 15 minutes and rinse with water. Use it twice per week.

Clearer Skin

Apple cider vinegar is also an effective all-natural astringent. It restores your body's pH level to normal which prevents future damage to your skin. Also, the acid in ACV absorbs excess oil, reduces your fine lines and makes your skin smoother. Soak washcloth in diluted apple cider vinegar and apply it on your face. You can also soak a cotton ball in diluted apple cider vinegar and dab it on your pimples, acne scars and age spots. Leave overnight to reduce their appearance.

Warts Remover

To get rid of unsightly warts naturally, soak a cotton ball in ACV and secure it in the affected area with a band-aid. You may also use a soaked gauze bandage in ACV and secure it in the affected area. This method is very effective and does not leave scars. Plus, it's pain-free.

Skin Toner

Apple cider vinegar is a great skin firming toner. Add ¼ cup ACV to ¾ cup distilled water and store in an air-tight container. Keep the mixture refrigerated. Apply the mixture to your face using a cotton ball right after you shower. The vinegar smell will disappear after it dries out.

Bad Breath Control

ACV helps kill odor-causing bacteria in the mouth that causes bad breath. Add one tablespoon of ACV in one cup of warm water and use it to gargle after brushing. For best results, gargle before going to bed at night. Rinse your mouth with water after gargling to prevent the acid in ACV from affecting your tooth enamel.

Whiter Teeth

ACV helps get rid of bacteria in the mouth, removes stains and whitens teeth. Combine 1 part apple cider vinegar to two parts water and swish it around your mouth. For better whitening effect, you can replace your toothpaste with baking soda instead. Rinse your mouth with water after gargling to prevent the acid in ACV from affecting your tooth enamel.

Aftershave

Whatever part of your body you shave, just use ACV solution to soothe your skin. Mix one part apple cider vinegar to 2 parts water and apply it on your shaved skin just as you would an aftershave lotion. Don't worry about the smell; it will dissipate when the vinegar has dried out.

Vaginal Douche

Apple Cider Vinegar helps keep your sensitive part down there smelling fresh and bacteria-free. The acetic acid in ACV restores the natural pH balance in your vagina, which prevents bad bacteria from building up. Dilute 2 tablespoons Apple Cider Vinegar in 1 liter of water. Use in the morning, during your bath and in the evening before going to bed.

Alternative Shampoo

For smoother, shinier hair without chemicals, simply mix 1 tablespoon ACV with one cup of water. Use it to rinse your hair as usual. Follow with a mixture of 1 tablespoon baking soda mixed in 1 cup of water. No need to shampoo.

Facial

For that radiant glow you've always wanted, the miracle vinegar is what you need.

Mix 1 tablespoon ACV in 1 cup of water. Wash your face with warm water. Do not apply soap, just plain warm water. Soak a clean cloth in warm water and wring excess water. Use this to cover your face for 3 minutes. Do this twice a week.

Do not use undiluted apple cider vinegar on sensitive skin. Other vinegars should not be used for these purposes as they are different from ACV.

Chapter 4: Apple Cider Vinegar Recipes

Now that you have learned the many benefits of apple cider vinegar, it is great to know that there are a lot of ACV recipes which you can use for various purposes.

Learn these easy apple cider vinegar recipes for your everyday needs.

ACV Detox Tea

Ingredients:

2 tablespoons Apple Cider Vinegar
1 tablespoon Raw Honey
1 cup Hot Water
Lemon squeeze
Dash of Cinnamon

Directions:

1. Pour some hot water in your mug.

2. Mix in ACV, lemon squeeze, cinnamon and honey. Mix thoroughly until all ingredients are well-combined.

3. Take a few deep breaths and sip while hot.

4. This concoction is great for detoxifying the gall bladder, balance blood sugar, enhance fat burning and aids in better digestion.

Apple Cider Energy Booster

Ingredients:

2 tablespoons Apple Cider Vinegar (unpasteurized, unfiltered)
1 teaspoon Maple Syrup
2 cups Natural Sparkling Water
Ice Cubes

Directions:

Mix all ingredients in a glass of water. Stir well and drink in the morning for that needed energy boost.

Always rinse your mouth with water if you take ACV in between meals or before going to bed to prevent prolonged contact on the enamel of your teeth.

Weight Loss Tea

Ingredients:

3 teaspoons Apple Cider Vinegar
2 teaspoons Honey
1 sachet Chamomile Tea
Dash of Cinnamon
1 cup of Hot Water

Directions:

1. Place Chamomile tea in the cup of hot water as usual.
2. Stir in honey, ACV and cinnamon.

Take this drink three times a day, before each meal.

Hair Tonic

Ingredients:

1 cup Apple Cider Vinegar
2 sprigs Rosemary, chopped
5 drops Lavender Essential Oil
5 cups Warm Water

Directions:

1. Pour the apple cider vinegar in a jar with a large lid. Add water until just below the lid. Mix thoroughly.
2. Store in a dry, cool area for one week.
3. Transfer in a lager container and dilute mixture in 3 cups of warm water. Stir in lavender essential oil. Mix thoroughly.
4. Transfer in a spray container and use as hair tonic for healthier, shinier hair. Use conditioner only when needed.

Always shake the spray container before every use. If your hair is color-treated, this tonic might affect your hair color. Consult with your hair stylist before using.

Candida Diet ACV Salad Dressing

Ingredients:

½ cup Apple Cider Vinegar
1 cup Olive Oil
2 tablespoons Dijon Mustard
1 teaspoon Onion Powder
1teaspoon Dried Thyme
1 teaspoon Dried Basil
3 cloves Garlic, minced
1 teaspoon Salt

Directions:

1. Add all ingredients in a container or bottle and shake well until ingredients are fully incorporated.
2. Store in the refrigerator when not in use.

Apple Cider Weight Loss Salad

Ingredients:

2 large Tomatoes, diced
2 medium Cucumbers, diced
¼ cup Apple Cider Vinegar
¼ cup Water
2 Spring Onions, diced
3 tablespoons Sugar
¼ teaspoon Black Pepper
¼ teaspoon Salt

Directions:

1. In a salad bowl, mix all ingredients together.
2. Put salad mix in an airtight container and store in the refrigerator for up to 7 days.

This vegetable salad is a great side dish or toppings for chicken, pork and fish dishes. It's great for peas and beans too.

Apple Cider Vinegar Health Drink

Ingredients:

1 tablespoon Apple Cider Vinegar
1 tablespoon Organic Coconut Oil
1 tablespoon Manuka Honey
1 teaspoon Tumeric Powder
4 drops Wild Oregano Oil

Directions:

1. In a small pot, melt coconut oil, turmeric powder and Manuka honey over low heat.
2. Remove from heat and stir in apple cider vinegar and oil of wild oregano.
3. Cool and add pear juice, pineapple juice or any juice of your choice.

This drink is also great for upset stomach, flatulence, colds and flu.

Oxymel Shots

Ingredients:

1 tablespoon Apple Cider Vinegar
2 tablespoons Water
1 tablespoon organic Apple Juice
1 tablespoon Honey

Directions:

1. Mix all ingredients in a small cup or shot glass.
2. Drink it just like you would do "shot" once in the morning.

Oxymel is an ancient Greek drink made from old wine (vinegar), honey and water. You can add ice cubes into this drink if you want it cold.

ACV Iced Tea

Ingredients:

2 tablespoons ACV
4 teaspoons raw Honey
1 teaspoon Cinnamon
1 cup of Hot Water

Directions:

1. In a small pot, heat a little water and add cinnamon. Simmer for 20 minutes.
2. In a cup, mix apple cider vinegar with honey, cinnamon mixture and purified water. Add some ice and enjoy a healthy, refreshing drink.

Drink this every morning and reap all the benefits of apple cider vinegar.

Sleep Enhancer

Ingredients:

2 tablespoons Apple Cider Vinegar
1 tablespoon Blackstrap Molasses
1 tablespoon Organic Honey
1 cup Warm Water

Directions:

1. Mix all ingredients in a cup of warm water.
2. Drink in the evening before you go to bed and feel fully refreshed the next morning.

You can also drink this recipe early in the morning to give you an energy boost that will help you go through your entire day.

Pick-Me-Up Apple Cider Vinegar Cocktail

Ingredients:

2 tablespoons Apple Cider Vinegar
1 glass Purified Water
2 teaspoons Organic Honey or 100% Maple Syrup

Directions:

Mix all ingredients in a glass of water. You can drink it with hot water or add some ice cubes if you want it cold.

You can add one more teaspoon of honey if you want it sweeter. This drink should be taken in the morning upon waking up, before eating lunch and before going to bed at night.

Healthy Salad Dressing

Ingredients:

1/2cup Organic Apple Cider Vinegar
1 tablespoon Raw Honey
½ teaspoon Liquid Aminos
1/3 cup Olive Oil blended with Sesame oil, Macadamia Oil or Flaxseed Oil
1 tablespoon Italian herbs

Directions:

1. Blend all ingredients in a blender and place in an air-tight container.
2. Store in the fridge up to 7 days.

This salad dressing is not only tasty but also very healthy. It goes well with most meat dishes and vegetable salads.

Fluffier Rice

Ingredients:

Rice
1 to 2 tablespoons Apple Cider Vinegar

Directions:

1. Cook rice as usual.
2. Sprinkle ACV while boiling.

Adding ACV on rice water will make the rice whiter and fluffier.

Chapter 5: ACV for Household Use

Although Apple Cider Vinegar is more expensive compared to other types of vinegar, when you think of all its benefits, it's actually very practical.

With ACV, you can keep your house clean, deodorized and germ-free without using chemicals that can be harmful to you and the environment. The acetic acid found in apple cider vinegar effectively cuts through grease and is also a very good deodorizer. It also has antifungal and antibacterial properties which prevent bacteria and molds from growing.

Why spend dollars on different household cleansers when you can get all these benefits in one all-natural product? Read on to learn more about the use of ACV for household cleaning.

Drain Declogger

Ingredients:

½ cup Apple Cider Vinegar
½ cup Baking Soda
½ cup Salt

Directions:

1. Mix baking soda and salt in a bowl and pour down your clogged drain.
2. Pour the apple cider vinegar and leave for 2 to 3 hours.
3. The baking soda and ACV will react and let go of a harmless gas.
4. Flush the drain with water.

Non-Toxic Floor Cleaner

Ingredients:

1.5 liters warm water

1 cup Apple Cider Vinegar

Directions:

1. Mix all ingredients together in a large pail.
2. Soak mop in the mixture and wring excess liquid.
3. Make sure to mop excess water from the floor to prevent warping on your tiles or wood floor.

All-Natural Kitchen Cleaner

Ingredients:

1 cup undiluted Apple Cider Vinegar
1cup 3% Solution Hydrogen Peroxide

Directions:

1   Fill your spray container with undiluted apple cider vinegar and spray it on your kitchen worktop and cutting boards.
2   Spray the surface right away with hydrogen peroxide.
3   Rinse the area with water and wipe dry.

ACV Bathroom Cleaner

Ingredients:

Undiluted, raw Apple Cider Vinegar
Baking Soda

Directions:

1. Place Apple Cider Vinegar in a spray bottle. Spray your entire bathroom, giving more attention to dirty areas and mould.
2. Sprinkle baking soda on the entire surface.
3. Leave for 2 to 3 hours.
4. Rinse with water. Spray remaining dirt and stains with ACV and scrub for a gleaming, odor-free bathroom.

House Deodorizer

Ingredients:

1 cup undiluted Apple Cider Vinegar
1 pail (bucket) of water

Directions:

1. Mix apple cider vinegar to the pail of water.
2. Soak cloth or mop in the mixture and use it to clean your entire household.
3. ACV breaks down volatile compounds in the air and kills germs and bacteria that cause the odor.

Apple cider vinegar has been touted by many as the "Miracle Cure" due to the multiple benefits that it offers. Aside from making dishes tastier, ACV is also used to cure various medical conditions, for beauty purposes and for household cleaning.

All-Purpose Cleaner

Ingredients:

1 cup raw Apple Cider Vinegar
1 cup Water
20 drops Citrus Essential Oil (or your preference)

Directions:

1. Combine all ingredients in a spray container.
2. Use it to clean surfaces, glass windows and furniture.
3. Always dry surface with cloth.
4. Shake container well before every use.

Chapter 6: ACV A Closer Look

Now that you know the many benefits of Apple Cider Vinegar (ACV), it is only right for you to know what makes it such a great product.

An organic, raw, ACV is made from organic apples that went through double fermentation. The fermentation process is responsible for the production of enzymes and preserves the health-promoting properties of apples.

What nutrients are found in raw, undiluted, Apple Cider Vinegar?

Acetic Acid – It prevents growth of bacteria and slows down the digestion of starch. This is why ACV is an effective aid in weight loss.

Ash - Helps the body maintain a healthy alkaline state.

Calcium - Helps build stronger teeth and bones. ACV diluted in water is an effective mouthwash and teeth whitener.

Enzymes -The enzymes found in apple cider vinegar boosts chemical reactions in the body, making fat burning faster.

Iron - Supports better blood health.

Magnesium - Supports heart health.

Malic Acid - Prevents germs, bacteria and fungus from contaminating the vinegar.

Pectin – Regulates cholesterol and blood pressure.

Potassium - Boosts organ and cellular functions.

Apple Cider Vinegar also contains numerous antioxidants such as Riboflavin, Thiamin and Niacin including Lycopene, Beta-carotene and Pantothenic Acid. These antioxidants rid the body of free radicals that destroys cells. Damaged cells causes a lot of medical conditions and they can potentially become cancer cells.

Furthermore, raw ACV contains the "mother" also known as Mycoderma Aceti which naturally develops during fermentation. Mother contains numerous friendly bacteria and living nutrients that are much needed for a well-balanced health.

If your body's pH level is not balanced, you will be more prone sickness and diseases. Acidity in the body leads to mineral loss in the bones, tissues, cells and organs. As a result, your vitamin absorption will be greatly affected. This will lead to easier build up of toxins and pathogens in your body and your immune system will be compromised.

All of these conditions can be prevented and cured by Apple Cider Vinegar. It is all-natural and its benefits have been proven for centuries. Even the Greek philosopher Hipocrates used Apple Cider Vinegar to heal infections.

There is no doubt. You should have a bottle or two of Apple Cider Vinegar in your kitchen and in your medicine cabinet. With all its benefits and uses, Apple Cider Vinegar deserves to be considered a "miracle cure". Not only does it cure a number of medical conditions, it also cures household odors and leaves your home squeaky clean. Best of all, ACV is also a great beauty partner for men and women of all ages.

Using Apple Cider Vinegar is very easy. Its either you use it as it is or dilute it in water. You may add some natural sweeteners if you prefer. Even so, Apple Cider Vinegar recipes do not require extensive steps and hard-to-find ingredients. Most of them are already present in your kitchen.

If you come to think of it, this multi-purpose vinegar is not really expensive. Instead of buying household cleaning products and deodorizers separately, all you need is Apple Cider Vinegar. So, you get to save more in the end. Plus, ACV is natural so it causes no harm to the environment. If you are going green, Apple Cider for your home is the right way to go.

Conclusion

In today's world, commercial products dominate the market. These products are sold cheaper only because they are made from cheap materials. Most, if not all of them, contains preservatives and harmful chemicals that can damage your health.

Natural products like Apple Cider Vinegar, on the other hand, hardly make it to grocery shops and food stores due to expensive costs. This is because organic, raw materials need more time and effort to grow. Plus, organic farmers are oftentimes not given enough attention by the government, forcing them to raise their prices to compensate their costs.

Even so, natural products are still healthier and safer to the body. If you want to rid your body of toxins and cure imbalances and various medical conditions, Apple Cider Vinegar will be your best friend. Once you have experienced the healing benefits of ACV, you will never again use any commercial products, no matter how cheap they are being sold.

In this book, you learned why Apple Cider Vinegar is such a great product. This book outlined the nutrients and minerals found in ACV and explained why and how it can cure diseases. You also learned various ACV recipes for health, beauty and home.

If you want to live a healthier life and get rid of diseases, going natural is the best way to go. Apple Cider Vinegar is made from natural ingredients and underwent natural fermentation processes. It does not contain anything that can harm your health. Instead, it contains healthy enzymes and bacteria that can help boost your immunity, keep your skin and body healthy and keep your household clean and deodorized.

The money you spent for this all-purpose vinegar is nothing compared to the numerous benefits you reap from it. It is about time to swap your ordinary vinegars to Apple Cider Vinegar.

I hope you enjoyed this book and hopefully, you can help your friends live a healthier life by sharing your experience with them.

Bonus Content

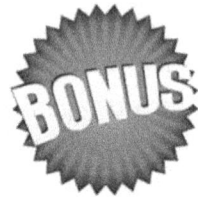

As a token of our appreciation Grand Reveur Publications would like to give you access to our exclusive bonus content (including free eBooks!).

Exclusive pre-release access to our latest eBooks

Free Grand Reveur eBooks during promotional periods.

A method ANYONE can use to publish their own book and make passive income

To receive bonus content please visit the following web site:

https://ignorelimits.leadpages.net/grandreveur publications/

As this is a limited time offer it would be a shame to miss out, I recommend grabbing these bonuses as soon as possible.

www.ingramcontent.com/pod-product-compliance
Lightning Source LLC
Chambersburg PA
CBHW070504290526
45790CB00003B/1094